Roger T. Blow

How to avoid vertigo with ease

Overcoming Vertigo

Vertigo

Copyright © by **Roger T. Blow** 2024. All rights reserved.

Before this document is duplicated or reproduced in any manner, the publisher's consent must be gained. Therefore, the contents within can neither be stored electronically, transferred, nor kept in a database. Neither in Part nor full can the document be copied, scanned, faxed, or retained without approval from the publisher or creator.

Vertigo

Table of Content

Introduction

Chapter 1

Chapter 2

Chapter 3

Chapter 4

Chapter 5

Chapter 6

Chapter 7

Chapter 8

Chapter 9

Introduction

Vertigo is a sensation of dizziness or a feeling that the environment around you is spinning or moving when it's not. It can be caused by various factors such as inner ear problems, certain medications, or underlying health conditions. It's often associated with symptoms like nausea, vomiting, and difficulty maintaining balance. If you experience vertigo frequently or severely, it's important to see a healthcare professional for proper diagnosis and treatment.

Chapter 1

Types of vertigo

1. Benign Paroxysmal Positional Vertigo (BPPV)

- BPPV is the most common cause of vertigo, accounting for approximately 20-30% of vertigo cases.

- It is characterized by brief episodes of intense vertigo triggered by specific head movements or changes in head position, such as rolling over in bed or looking up.

- BPPV occurs due to the displacement of small calcium carbonate crystals (otoconia) within the inner ear, specifically the semicircular canals, leading to abnormal sensations of motion.

- Diagnosis is typically made through a physical examination and confirmed with positional tests such as the Dix-Hallpike maneuver.

Vertigo

- Treatment often involves canalith repositioning maneuvers, such as the Epley maneuver or Semont maneuver, which aim to reposition the displaced crystals and alleviate symptoms.

2. Meniere's Disease
- Meniere's disease is a chronic inner ear disorder characterized by a serious and recurrent episodes of vertigo, fluctuating hearing impairment or loss, tinnitus (ringing in the ears), and a sensation of fullness or pressure in the affected or the hurting ear.
- The exact cause of Meniere's disease is not fully understood but is believed to involve abnormalities in the fluid balance within the inner ear.
- Diagnosis is based on a combination of symptoms, medical history, and audiometric testing.
- Treatment may include dietary modifications (reducing salt intake), medications to control symptoms (diuretics, vestibular suppressants), and in severe cases, surgical procedures such as

endolymphatic sac decompression or vestibular nerve section.

3. Vestibular Neuritis

- Vestibular neuritis is an inflammatory disorder or a critical disorder affecting and destructing the vestibular nerve, which connects the inner ear to the brainstem.
- It typically presents with sudden onset of severe vertigo, often accompanied by nausea, vomiting, and imbalance, but without hearing loss or tinnitus.
- Vestibular neuritis is commonly caused by viral infections, such as herpes simplex virus or varicella-zoster virus.
- Diagnosis is based on clinical presentation, medical history, and vestibular function tests.
- Treatment may include medications to alleviate symptoms (antihistamines, antiemetics) and vestibular rehabilitation therapy to promote compensation and recovery of balance function.

Vertigo

4. Migrainous Vertigo

- Migrainous vertigo, also known as vestibular migraine or migrainous vestibulopathy, refers to vertigo or dizziness that occurs in association with migraine headaches.

- It is characterized by recurrent episodes of vertigo lasting minutes to hours, often accompanied by headache, photophobia (sensitivity to light), phonophobia (sensitivity to sound), and visual disturbances.

- The exact mechanisms underlying migrainous vertigo are not fully understood but are believed to involve interactions between the vestibular system and migraine pathways in the brain.

- Diagnosis is based on a history of migraine headaches and characteristic vestibular symptoms, often supported by ruling out other potential causes of vertigo.

- Treatment may involve migraine preventive medications, lifestyle modifications, and management of acute vertigo symptoms with vestibular suppressants or antiemetics.

These different types of vertigo have distinct characteristics, underlying causes, diagnostic approaches, and treatment strategies. Understanding the specific type of vertigo is crucial for proper management and improving quality of life for individuals experiencing these symptoms.

Chapter 2

Causes of vertigo

1. Inner ear issues: Problems with the inner ear, such as benign paroxysmal positional vertigo (BPPV), labyrinthitis, or vestibular neuritis, can lead to vertigo.

2. Meniere's disease: This condition affects the inner ear and can cause episodes of vertigo along with hearing loss, ringing in the ears (tinnitus), and a feeling of fullness in the ear.

3. Migraines: Some people experience vertigo as a symptom of migraines, known as vestibular migraines.

4. Head injuries: Traumatic head injuries or concussions can damage the inner ear or the balance centers in the brain, leading to vertigo.

5. Medications: Certain medications, particularly those that affect the inner ear or brain function, can cause vertigo as a side effect.

6. Anxiety disorders: Anxiety and panic attacks can sometimes cause symptoms of vertigo or feelings of dizziness.

7. Brainstem or cerebellar disorders: Conditions affecting the brainstem or cerebellum, such as stroke, multiple sclerosis, or tumors, can disrupt the balance centers and cause vertigo.

8. Dehydration or low blood pressure: Changes in fluid levels or blood pressure can affect the inner ear and lead to vertigo.

9. Ear infections: Infections in the inner ear or middle ear can cause inflammation and disrupt balance, leading to vertigo.

10. Aging: As people age, changes in the inner ear and other systems involved in balance can increase the risk of experiencing vertigo.

These are just a few examples, and there may be other causes as well. It's important to consult with a healthcare professional for proper diagnosis and treatment if you experience vertigo.

Chapter 3

Risk factors of experiencing vertigo

1. Age: Vertigo becomes more common as people age, as age-related changes in the inner ear and balance systems can increase the risk.

2. Inner ear disorders: Conditions such as benign paroxysmal positional vertigo (BPPV), Meniere's disease, and vestibular neuritis can predispose individuals to vertigo.

3. Head injuries: Traumatic head injuries or concussions can damage the inner ear or the balance centers in the brain, increasing the risk of vertigo.

4. Certain medications: Some medications, particularly those that affect the inner ear or brain function, can cause vertigo as a side effect.

Vertigo

5. Migraines: Individuals with a history of migraines, especially vestibular migraines, have an increased risk of experiencing vertigo.

6. Anxiety and stress: Anxiety disorders and stress can sometimes trigger or exacerbate symptoms of vertigo.

7. Smoking: Smoking has been linked to an increased risk of developing inner ear disorders, such as Meniere's disease, which can lead to vertigo.

8. Alcohol consumption: Excessive alcohol consumption can affect the inner ear and disrupt balance, increasing the risk of vertigo.

9. Dehydration: Inadequate fluid intake can lead to dehydration, which can affect the inner ear and increase the risk of vertigo.

10. Family history: Some individuals may have a genetic predisposition to certain inner ear disorders or conditions that can cause vertigo.

These are just a few examples of risk factors for vertigo. It's essential to be aware of these factors and take steps to minimize risk, such as avoiding known triggers and maintaining overall health and wellness. If you experience frequent or severe vertigo, it's important to consult with a healthcare professional for proper evaluation and management.

Chapter 4

Methods of Diagnosing vertigo

1. Medical history: Your doctor will ask about your symptoms, including when they started, how long they last, what triggers them, and any associated symptoms like hearing loss or ringing in the ears (tinnitus).

2. Physical examination: This may include checking your balance, eye movements, and neurological function. Your doctor may perform the Dix-Hallpike maneuver or other positional tests to assess for certain types of vertigo, such as benign paroxysmal positional vertigo (BPPV).

3. Vestibular function tests: These tests evaluate the function of the inner ear and vestibular system.

Common tests include electronystagmography, videonystagmography , and rotary chair testing.

4. Imaging studies: In some cases, imaging tests such as magnetic resonance imaging (MRI) or computed tomography (CT) scans may be ordered to rule out structural abnormalities in the brain or inner ear.

5. Blood tests: Blood tests may be performed to check for underlying conditions that could be contributing to vertigo, such as infections or metabolic disorders.

6. Electroencephalogram (EEG): In some cases, an EEG may be used to evaluate brain function and rule out conditions such as epilepsy that can cause symptoms similar to vertigo.

7. Audiometric testing: Hearing tests may be conducted to assess for hearing loss or other auditory problems that could be related to vertigo.

The specific tests ordered will depend on your individual symptoms and medical history. It's important to consult with a healthcare professional for proper diagnosis and management of vertigo.

Chapter 5

Common symptoms associated with vertigo

Vertigo is a sensation of spinning or motion when there is no actual movement. It is often or usually accompanied or comes along by other severe symptoms that can vary in severity and duration.

1. Dizziness: Vertigo is characterized by a feeling of dizziness or lightheadedness, as if the world around you is spinning or tilting. This sensation can be disorienting and unsettling, leading to a loss of balance and coordination.

2. Spinning Sensations: Individuals experiencing vertigo may describe sensations of spinning, whirling, or rotating, even when they are sitting or lying still. These sensations can be brief or prolonged and may worsen with certain head movements.

3. Nausea and Vomiting: Vertigo often triggers feelings of nausea, sometimes accompanied by vomiting. The sensation of spinning or imbalance can disrupt the normal functioning of the vestibular system and lead to gastrointestinal discomfort.

4. Imbalance: A sense of imbalance or unsteadiness is common during vertigo episodes. Individuals may feel as though they are swaying, tilting, or about to fall, even when standing still. This can increase or multiply the risk of falls and accidents.

5. Visual Disturbances: Vertigo may be associated with visual disturbances such as blurring, double vision, or difficulty focusing. These visual symptoms can exacerbate feelings of dizziness and contribute to disorientation.

6. Sweating and Pallor: Some individuals may experience sweating, clamminess, or a pale complexion during vertigo episodes. These autonomic symptoms can accompany the sensation of dizziness and contribute to overall discomfort.

7. Anxiety and Panic: Vertigo episodes can be frightening and may trigger feelings of anxiety or panic in some individuals. Fear of falling or losing control can exacerbate symptoms and lead to further distress.

It's important to note that the symptoms of vertigo can vary depending on the underlying cause and individual factors. While some people may experience mild and occasional vertigo episodes, others may have severe and recurrent symptoms that significantly impact their daily lives. If you experience frequent or severe vertigo symptoms, it's

Vertigo

important to seek medical evaluation to determine the underlying cause and appropriate treatment.

Chapter 6

Treatment options for vertigo

1. Vestibular Rehabilitation Therapy (VRT)

- VRT is a specialized exercise-based program designed to improve balance and reduce symptoms of vertigo.

- It involves a series of exercises and activities aimed at promoting adaptation, habituation, and compensation of the vestibular system.

- VRT is tailored to each individual's specific symptoms and functional limitations and is typically conducted under the guidance of a trained physical therapist.

- The exercises may include gaze stabilization exercises, balance training, habituation exercises to desensitize the vestibular system to motion, and specific maneuvers to promote compensation.

2. Medication

- Medications may be prescribed to alleviate symptoms of vertigo and associated nausea and vomiting.

- Vestibular suppressants such as antihistamines (e.g., meclizine, dimenhydrinate) and benzodiazepines (e.g., diazepam, lorazepam) may be used to reduce dizziness and motion sickness.

- Antiemetic medications such as promethazine or ondansetron may be prescribed to alleviate nausea and vomiting.

- In cases of migrainous vertigo, migraine preventive medications such as beta-blockers, calcium channel blockers, or tricyclic antidepressants may be used to reduce the frequency and severity of vertigo attacks.

3. Canalith Repositioning Maneuvers

- Canalith repositioning maneuvers, also known as particle repositioning maneuvers, are a series of specific head and body movements designed to reposition displaced calcium carbonate crystals (otoconia) in the inner ear.

- The most well-known maneuver is the Epley maneuver, which is used to treat benign paroxysmal positional vertigo (BPPV) affecting the posterior semicircular canal.

- Other maneuvers, such as the Semont maneuver or Brandt-Daroff exercises, may be used to treat different types of BPPV or to facilitate adaptation and habituation of the vestibular system.

4. Lifestyle Changes

- Lifestyle modifications may help manage vertigo symptoms and reduce the frequency of vertigo episodes.

- Avoiding triggers such as caffeine, alcohol, tobacco, and certain medications that can exacerbate vertigo.

- Maintaining adequate hydration and a balanced diet to support overall health and vestibular function.
- Practicing stress-reduction techniques such as relaxation exercises, mindfulness, and deep breathing to minimize stress and anxiety, which can exacerbate vertigo symptoms.

5. Surgical Interventions

- In severe cases of vertigo that do not respond to conservative treatments, surgical interventions may be considered.
- Surgical procedures such as vestibular nerve section or labyrinthectomy may be performed to selectively ablate or remove the vestibular organs, thereby reducing or eliminating vertigo symptoms.
- These surgical interventions are typically reserved for cases of disabling vertigo that significantly impair quality of life and have failed to respond to other treatment modalities.

Vertigo

It's important to note that the choice of treatment for vertigo depends on the underlying cause, severity of symptoms, individual preferences, and response to previous treatments. A comprehensive evaluation by a healthcare professional is essential to determine the most appropriate treatment plan for each individual.

Chapter 7

How vertigo can impact quality of life and strategies for coping with vertigo-related challenges

1. Work Life

- Vertigo can interfere with concentration, productivity, and performance at work, particularly in tasks that require focus and balance.

- Individuals with vertigo may experience difficulty working in environments with visual or motion stimuli, such as on a computer screen or in a busy office.

- Severe vertigo episodes may necessitate time off work or adjustments to work schedules, leading to absenteeism or decreased work efficiency.

- Strategies for coping with vertigo at work may include requesting accommodations such as flexible hours, ergonomic adjustments, or telecommuting options to minimize triggers and accommodate symptom fluctuations.

2. Social Activities

- Vertigo can impact participation in social activities, leisure pursuits, and recreational sports that involve movement or visual stimuli.

- Fear of vertigo episodes or embarrassment about potential loss of balance in public settings may lead to social withdrawal and isolation.

- Individuals with vertigo may feel anxious or self-conscious in social situations, leading to avoidance of social gatherings or events.

- Strategies for coping with vertigo in social settings may include communicating openly with friends and family about vertigo symptoms, identifying supportive social networks, and choosing activities that are less likely to trigger symptoms.

3. Mental Well-being

- Vertigo can have a significant impact on mental well-being, leading to feelings of frustration, anxiety, depression, and decreased self-esteem.

- Chronic vertigo symptoms can erode confidence and self-efficacy, affecting overall quality of life and sense of independence.

- The unpredictability of vertigo episodes and their disruptive effects on daily activities can contribute to feelings of loss of control and helplessness.

- Strategies for coping with vertigo-related mental health challenges may include seeking professional support from therapists or counselors, practicing relaxation techniques such as deep breathing or mindfulness meditation, and engaging in activities that promote stress reduction and emotional resilience.

4. Coping Strategies

Vertigo

- Educating oneself about vertigo and its triggers, symptoms, and management strategies can empower individuals to better cope with their condition.

- Developing a personalized vertigo management plan in collaboration with healthcare professionals can help individuals identify effective coping strategies and treatment options.

- Engaging in regular physical activity, such as vestibular rehabilitation exercises, yoga, or tai chi, can improve balance, reduce symptoms, and enhance overall well-being.

- Adopting healthy lifestyle habits, such as maintaining a balanced diet, staying hydrated, getting adequate sleep, and managing stress, can help minimize vertigo symptoms and improve overall quality of life.

Overall, vertigo can pose significant challenges to daily functioning and well-being, but with proper support, education, and coping strategies,

Vertigo

individuals can learn to manage their symptoms effectively and maintain an active and fulfilling life. It's important for individuals with vertigo to seek support from healthcare professionals, friends, and family members to navigate the challenges of living with this condition.

Chapter 8

Prevention and management strategies for vertigo

1. Avoiding Triggers

- Identify and avoid known triggers that can exacerbate vertigo episodes. Common triggers may include certain foods (e.g., caffeine, alcohol, salty foods), stress, fatigue, sudden head movements, and visual stimuli.

- Keep a journal to track vertigo episodes and potential triggers, allowing for better identification and avoidance of triggers in the future.

2. Staying Hydrated

- Dehydration can worsen vertigo symptoms, so it's important to stay hydrated by drinking an adequate amount of water throughout the day.

- Avoid excessive consumption of caffeine and alcohol, as they can contribute to dehydration and trigger vertigo.

3. Practicing Stress-Reduction Techniques
- Stress and anxiety can exacerbate or increase vertigo symptoms, so practicing stress-reduction techniques can be beneficial and important for avoid vertigo.
- Techniques such as deep breathing exercises, progressive muscle relaxation, meditation, and mindfulness can help reduce stress and promote relaxation, thereby minimizing vertigo symptoms.

4. Maintaining a Healthy Lifestyle
- Adopting a healthy lifestyle can help manage vertigo symptoms and improve overall well-being.
- Eat a balanced diet rich in fruits, vegetables, whole grains, and lean proteins to support overall health and vestibular function.

- Get regular exercise to improve balance, coordination, and overall fitness. Activities such as walking, swimming, yoga, and tai chi can be particularly beneficial for individuals with vertigo.

- Prioritize adequate sleep to support optimal physical and mental health. Establish a good regular sleep schedule and create a relaxing bedtime routine to promote restful sleep and avoid mental stress.

5. Vestibular Rehabilitation Therapy (VRT)

- VRT is a specialized exercise program designed to improve balance, reduce dizziness, and enhance overall vestibular function.

- Working with a trained physical therapist, individuals can learn specific exercises and techniques tailored to their unique symptoms and functional limitations.

- VRT aims to promote adaptation, habituation, and compensation of the vestibular system, helping

Vertigo

individuals better cope with vertigo symptoms and regain confidence in their balance and mobility.

6. Medication Management

- Follow your healthcare provider's recommendations regarding medication management for vertigo. This may include taking prescribed medications to alleviate symptoms or prevent vertigo attacks.

- Be aware of potential side effects of medications and communicate any concerns or adverse reactions to your healthcare provider.

By incorporating these prevention and management strategies into daily life, individuals with vertigo can minimize the frequency and severity of vertigo episodes, improve overall quality of life, and better cope with the challenges of living with this condition. It's vital and important to work closely with healthcare professionals to develop or build a

Vertigo

personalized treatment plan that addresses individual needs and goals.

Chapter 9

Advancements in vertigo research

1. Advancements in Diagnostic Techniques

- High-resolution imaging techniques such as magnetic resonance imaging (MRI) and computed tomography (CT) have enabled more detailed visualization of the inner ear structures and the vestibular system, facilitating accurate diagnosis of vestibular disorders.

- Technological advancements in vestibular function testing, including videonystagmography (VNG), rotary chair testing, and vestibular evoked myogenic potentials (VEMP), have improved the assessment of vestibular function and contributed to the differentiation of various types of vertigo.

2. Understanding of Underlying Mechanisms

- Research has deepened our understanding of the pathophysiology of vertigo, including the role of the vestibular system, central nervous system, and peripheral vestibular organs in the generation of vertigo symptoms.

- Studies have identified genetic predispositions and molecular pathways associated with certain vestibular disorders, providing insights into potential targets for novel therapies.

3. New Treatment Modalities

- Emerging treatments such as vestibular implants and neuromodulation techniques hold promise for individuals with severe or refractory vertigo who do not respond to conventional therapies.

- Pharmacological research has led to the development of targeted medications that address specific mechanisms underlying vertigo, including vestibular suppressants, migraine preventatives, and agents that modulate neurotransmitter activity in the vestibular system.

- Advances in vestibular rehabilitation therapy (VRT), including the incorporation of virtual reality technology and gamified exercises, have enhanced the effectiveness of rehabilitation programs and improved outcomes for individuals with vestibular disorders.

4. Telemedicine and Remote Monitoring

- The integration of telemedicine platforms and wearable sensor technologies has facilitated remote assessment and monitoring of vertigo symptoms, allowing for more frequent monitoring and timely interventions.

- Tele-rehabilitation programs have expanded access to vestibular rehabilitation services, particularly in underserved or remote areas, improving the availability and convenience of care for individuals with vertigo.

5. Multidisciplinary Collaborations

- Increasing collaboration between specialists in otolaryngology, neurology, physical therapy, and audiology has led to more comprehensive and integrated care approaches for individuals with vertigo.

- Multidisciplinary research consortia and networks have been established to foster collaboration, share best practices, and accelerate the translation of research findings into clinical practice.

These advancements hold promise for improving the diagnosis, treatment, and management of vertigo, ultimately enhancing the quality of life for individuals affected by this debilitating condition. Continued research efforts and interdisciplinary collaborations will be essential to further advance our understanding of vertigo and develop innovative therapies to address the diverse needs of patients.

www.ingramcontent.com/pod-product-compliance
Lightning Source LLC
Chambersburg PA
CBHW050249230526
45470CB00005B/2182